pin it!

Pin It!

20 fabulous bobby pin hairstyles

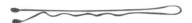

ANNAMARIE TENDLER

PHOTOGRAPHS BY JUSTIN OUELLETTE

CHRONICLE BOOKS
SAN FRANCISCO

Library of Congress Cataloging-in-Publication Data:

Names: Tendler, Annamarie, author.
Title: Pin it! : 20 fabulous bobby pin hairstyles / Annamarie Tendler ;
   photographs by Justin Ouellette.
Description: San Francisco : Chronicle Books, 2017. | Includes index.
Identifiers: LCCN 2016025897 | ISBN 9781452158389 (hardback)
Subjects: LCSH: Hairstyles. | Bobby pins. | Hairdressing—Equipment and supplies. |
   Handicraft for girls. | BISAC: CRAFTS & HOBBIES / Fashion. | HEALTH &
   FITNESS / Beauty & Grooming.
Classification: LCC TT976 .T46 2017 | DDC 646.7/24—dc23 LC record available
   at https://lccn.loc.gov/2016025897

Manufactured in China

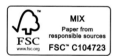

Design by Anne Kenady

Stylist: Maryssa Stumpf

10 9 8 7 6 5 4 3 2 1

Chronicle books and gifts are available at special quantity discounts to corpora-
tions, professional associations, literacy programs, and other organizations. For
details and discount information, please contact our corporate/premiums depart-
ment at corporatesales@chroniclebooks.com or at 1-800-759-0190.

Chronicle Books LLC
680 Second Street
San Francisco, California 94107
www.chroniclebooks.com

For my grandmother, Shirley, and my late grandmother, Lois—
two smart, strong, and stylish women.

CONTENTS

INTRODUCTION

Welcome to *Pin It!*, the ultimate bobby pin* hairstyling guide. Remember when bobby pins came in only three colors: black, brown, and blond? I do! Back then, whether to hold a perfectly tight ballet bun or to keep a highly questionable prom updo intact, the only job a bobby pin had *besides* keeping your hair together was to disappear and never be seen again. Well, the days of the boring bobby pin are over! Now you can find all sorts of colorful and fashionable pins that deserve to take center stage in your hairstyles. Use glitter pins in star formations to take your ponytail to another galaxy, or match bright pink pins to your lipstick for a next-level look. You can even decorate your own pins with paint, nail polish, or glitter.

So what exactly can you expect from this book? It doesn't matter if you have short hair or long hair, if you are a hairstyling expert or are hairstyling challenged, there is a bobby pin styling idea in *Pin It!* for you. For each look, I tell you exactly what tools you need to achieve it, the best hair length for the style, and the difficulty level. (And yes, don't worry: you'll find a lot of easy styles!) With the step-by-step instructions and photos, I've made these styles simple for anyone to re-create. If you're looking for creative ways to decorate your own pins, head to the back of the book for some fun DIY pin projects.

As you go through this book I urge you to be creative. Mix up the types of pins (ombré! glitter!) and switch up the designs (starbursts! chevrons!). Use any bobby pin technique with any hairstyle to create your own wearable art. *There are no rules.* Remember, this book is just a jumping-off point for the amazing and unique styles I know you can create.

Happy pinning!

*In some parts of the world these are called "hair grips" or "hair pins." I say "bobby pins"—just know I'm talking about those cute pins you see in the book's photos!

GETTING STARTED

TOOLS AND PRODUCTS

While the looks in this book are easy to achieve, there are some basic tools and helpful products you will need to get started; some are essential and others you may simply find helpful. Any of these tools can be found at a drugstore or beauty supply store. For each look I list the tools needed, but I've provided a full list on the following pages should you want to put together a tool kit ahead of time.

STYLING TOOLS

BOAR-BRISTLE HAIRBRUSH

This brush is used for smoothing hair and is especially great for creating a sleek ponytail or a bun.

BOBBY PINS, CONVENTIONAL

While all of the styles in this book showcase decorative pins, you'll want some conventional bobby pins on hand to secretly hold together parts of the hairstyles. Since they won't be a focal part of the styles, these pins should match the color of your hair. Found at any drugstore or beauty supply store, or online, these pins come in blond, brown, or black to match most hair tones.

BOBBY PINS, MINI

These are just like conventional pins but half the size and are great for creating more intricate designs. They also work well for holding thin, fine, or short hair.

CURLING WAND OR CURLING IRON

A curling iron and a curling wand are two different things: An iron has a clasp for holding the hair and a wand does not. An iron creates a more polished ringlet (which I feel is undesirable), and a wand creates loose waves (desirable!). The good news is that if you own only a curling iron, but you want to use it like a wand, you can—just ignore the clasp. I prefer a wand with a 1¼-in/3-cm barrel. If your hair is on the shorter side, you may find that a wand with a 1-in/2.5-cm barrel works best, since you have less hair to wrap around the wand.

> To use: Holding the end of a small (about 1 in/2.5 cm) section of your hair, wrap the section around the barrel of the wand or iron (ignore the clasp and wrap right around it) in the direction you want your hair to curl. Hold for 10 seconds and release.

FINE-TOOTHED COMB

This type of comb is perfect for parting your hair. It's usually step number 1 for any hairstyle.

FLAT IRON

You can use a flat iron to smooth out, straighten, or even curl hair. In general, the 1-in/2.5-cm flat iron works best. When curling my own hair, I often find that using a flat iron is easier and faster than using a curling iron. Try both methods and decide which works better for you.

> To flatten: Place the flat iron at the roots of a small (about 1 in/2.5 cm) section of your hair, and apply firm pressure as you move the iron down past the ends of your hair.

> To curl: Place the flat iron at the roots— or wherever you want the curl to start— of a small (about 1 in/2.5 cm) section of hair and move the iron down the hair shaft while also turning the iron in the direction you want the curl to go.

HAIR CLIPS

You'll need clips to hold back sections of hair while creating the styles. Crocodile clips or duckbill clips work best.

HAIR ELASTICS

The best elastics are those without any metal clasps. These help hold your hair in place without drooping or getting caught. I prefer the thick elastics, as they create a more bouncy ponytail, even in thinner hair. If your hair is very thin and fine, opt for thinner elastics.

HAIR ELASTICS, CLEAR

The clear elastics are perfect for holding the ends of braids where the hair is typically not very thick, and they seamlessly disappear into the style.

MIRROR

It is essential to be able to look into a mirror when doing these looks. For some looks you will need a mirror in front of you *and* behind you so you can see the back of your head. You can use a handheld mirror to check your placement, or if you have nifty bathroom mirrors that fold out, use those so you can see both the front and back of your head at the same time.

PADDLE BRUSH

Use to detangle wet hair after washing.

WIDE-TOOTHED COMB

This is the best tool for detangling wet curly hair.

STYLING PRODUCTS

BEACH SPRAY (SALT SPRAY)

This spray, which is literally made of salt water, adds texture and volume to hair.

> Best used for: creating tousled looks and beachy waves.

DRY SHAMPOO

This is a powder (usually found in spray form) that works well to absorb oil from hair.

> Best used for: absorbing oil and adding texture to second-day hair.

HAIR SPRAY

Creates a strong hold so hair stays put in your styles.

> Best used for: holding curls and finished styles, and smoothing down fly-aways.

LEAVE-IN CONDITIONER

This is just what it sounds like—a conditioner that you don't rinse out.

> Best used for: detangling wet hair and protecting the hair shaft during heat styling.

SERUM

This is an oil-based product meant to be applied to wet hair before styling.

> Best used for: creating shine and reducing frizz.

SHINE SPRAY

A finishing spray that, when applied lightly, adds a touch of shine to the hair.

> Best used for: misting over a finished style to create a layer of shine. To apply, hold the spray about half an arm's length away from your head so that just a light layer mists your hair.

TEXTURIZING SPRAY

Adds texture to hair, making it easier to grip and style. Almost every haircare company makes a texturizing spray; you just need to find your favorite.

> Best used for: adding texture to the hair before styling.

HAIRCARE TIPS

Now, you can't fit everyone's hair into the check boxes of straight, wavy, or curly. Some people have straight hair in front and wavy in back. Some people have tight curls; some have loose curls. Some have straight hair on top but then it gets all wavy underneath. There's so much variation! Whether your hair is fine or thick, curly or straight, the key to great-looking styles is keeping it healthy. On the following pages I've listed a few tips for maintaining your best hair.

BRAID

If you have long hair, a braid can be a powerful deterrent from tangling and breakage. I have very long hair, so I braid my hair before I go to sleep or if I'm outside on very windy days. If you do the same, you won't be working up a rat's nest while you sleep or battle the wind.

BRUSH

Brushing your hair stimulates your scalp and helps get rid of hair that has fallen out but is still hanging around in all your hair. Using a boar-bristle brush will evenly distribute the oil from your scalp down the hair shaft, which is basically like using a hair serum you don't have to pay for! If you have curly or kinky hair, brushing after the hair is dry and styled will disrupt the curl, so instead brush right before you shower.

LOWER THE HEAT

A lot of irons and wands come with temperature dials that allow you to control the heat. Do me a favor: Don't turn these all the way up to the highest setting! Leave those settings to your professional stylist. Heat styling can cause damage and breakage, and you can minimize this by keeping the iron on medium heat.

MOISTURIZE

Whether your hair is naturally frizzy every day or you find yourself in Louisiana in August, you can combat frizz with leave-in conditioners, hair serums, and oils (like argan oil). Choose products based on the texture and density of your hair—a good rule of thumb is using lighter products for thin hair or very fine hair, and something heavier for coarse or kinky hair. But I say try a bunch of products and find what works best for you!

TRIM

About every three to four months, trim your hair to keep hair ends healthy and to remove any split ends. It's especially important to get trims regularly if you style with heat often, as this can be hard on your hair.

WASH SPARINGLY

I don't wash my hair every day, and I don't think most people should. If you have very fine, very thin hair that gets greasy easily, then by all means, wash your hair as often as you need to. But for everyone else, I suggest stretching washes to at least every other day. I have fine, medium- to thick-density hair that is naturally wavy and curly, but I usually heat-style it. I wait two or three days between washings. *Maybe* I'll wash every other day if I have somewhere really important to go. Spreading out my washes also allows my blow dry (or curl, or straightening) to last longer.

Here's the thing about your scalp: The more you wash it, the more oil it's going to produce. So if you can get in the habit of spacing out your washes, you'll soon see that your hair won't get oily nearly as fast. If I get to the second day and I look at my shampoo and think, "Nah," I will brush my hair with a boar-bristle brush to distribute the oil evenly, and *then* I will use said oil to my advantage by pulling my hair into a super-sleek low bun. I keep brushing with the boar-bristle brush as I pull my hair into the bun. My hair looks shiny from the oil, and

because everything has been smoothed out, it looks expertly styled. (I have just divulged to you my greatest personal hairstyling secret; with great power comes great responsibility!)

TOO CLEAN TO STYLE?

Styling hair is actually easiest when hair is not 100 percent clean. Freshly washed hair is often too soft and slippery, making it difficult for braids, hair elastics, and pins to hold tightly. That said, greasy hair doesn't look good no matter what you do with it! I personally like to style with clean hair, but only after adding a good texturizing spray. This allows the roots to remain clean while giving hair the texture it needs to hold the style.

SPECIALTY PINS

Of course, you'll need specialty bobby pins to create these looks—
that's the whole point of this book! You can find decorative pins at
beauty stores or online, such as on Etsy.com, or you can easily make
them yourself. At the end of this book you will find five DIY projects
for decorating pins with just a few materials. The types of specialty
pins we use in this book include glitter, colored, ombré, and those
with ornamental details such as pearls or flowers. Flip through to get
a sense of the types of pins you'll want to use and then stock up (or
make your own!) before getting started on these looks.

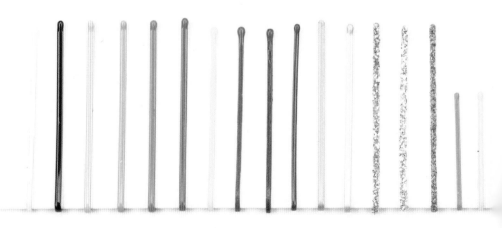

PINS TO PURCHASE

Although it's always more fun to make your own, I suggest stocking up on some specialty pins to use in addition to your handmade treasures.

White: Just like conventional pins but white in color, these pins are the perfect canvas for nail polish, because the white is easy to cover (see page 119).

High Gloss: These are just like conventional pins but with a high-gloss finish.

Ombré: This type comes in a set from light to dark. We use pink in this book, but other shades are available.

Metallic: A gold, silver, or bronze finish is applied to these conventional pins.

Glitter: These bobby pins are infused with flecks of sparkle glitter.

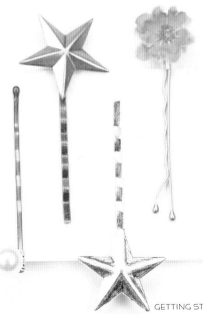

TOOLS AND MATERIALS FOR DIY PINS

Making fabulous pins is super easy with just a few basic craft materials on hand. Stock up before you get started.

ALUMINUM FOIL
Great to use to cover your craft space for easy cleanup and as a place for your glue.

EXTRA-FINE CRAFT GLITTER
Loose, very fine glitter generally sold in a jar.

HOT GLUE GUN
Hot glue is best for affixing flowers, beads, jewels, or other three-dimensional material to your pins.

INDEX CARDS OR FOLDED PAPER
Have these on hand to act as a holder for your pin while you craft. The paper allows you to paint or glue the pin without having to touch it.

NAIL POLISH
Use for painting pins different colors. It works best on blond or white bobby pins.

SCISSORS
Craft scissors are helpful for cutting jewelry wire and other materials.

SPONGE BRUSH
This is just like a paintbrush but with a sponge on the end; it's the best tool for applying glue to pins.

WHITE GLUE
Use as an adhesive base for glitter pins.

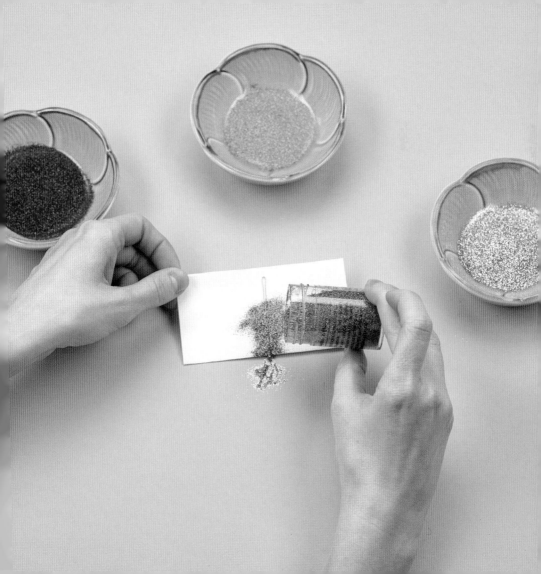

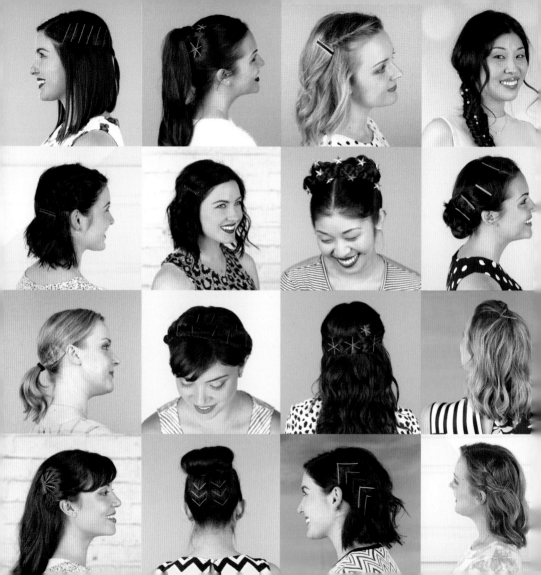

THE LOOKS

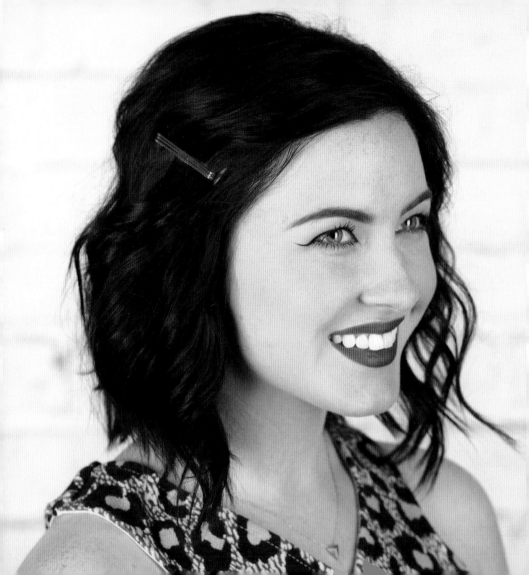

MATCH POINT

Match your pins to your pout for a perfectly polished look.

DIFFICULTY LEVEL

easy

IDEAL HAIR LENGTH

chin and longer

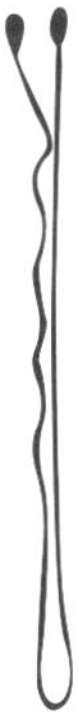

MATERIALS

fine-toothed comb

curling iron or curling wand

3 bright pink bobby pins

bright pink lipstick to match

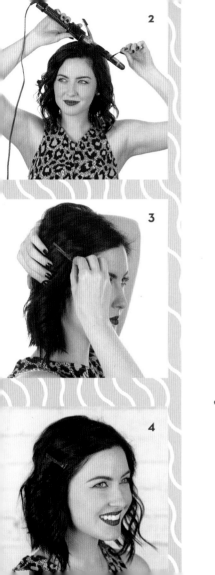

1. Use the comb to create a side part.

2. Loosely curl your hair all over using a curling iron or curling wand.

3. On the side opposite of your part, gently hold the hair with one hand, and with your other hand insert three bright pink bobby pins in the area between your temple and your ear so they are flush next to each other with no space between.

4. Apply lipstick to match your pink pins and go conquer the day!

STYLE TIP

Don't like pink? No problem! Make your own pins with any nail polish (see page 119) and match them to your favorite color lipstick.

If you're in a rush and don't have time to curl your hair, try this style with straight hair for a sleeker look.

STARBURST CROWN

Fill your head with stars in this fun yet elegant style that can dress up even the most casual look.

DIFFICULTY LEVEL

hard

IDEAL HAIR LENGTH

shoulder and longer

MATERIALS

fine-toothed comb

crocodile clip

conventional bobby pins to match your hair color

6 gold metallic bobby pins

3 gold glitter bobby pins

3 mini gold glitter bobby pins

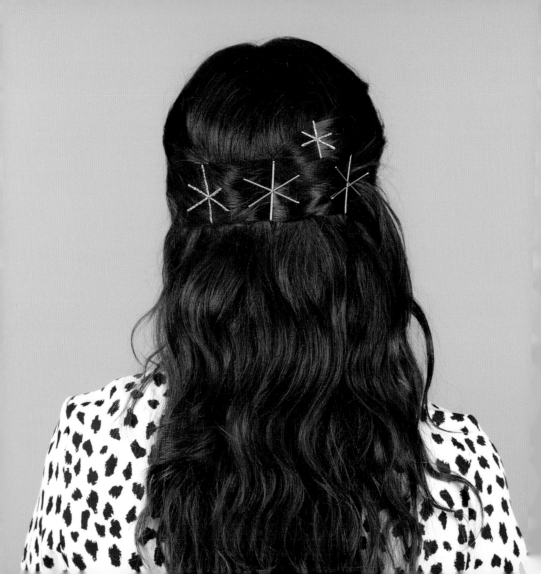

1. Using a comb, create a section from the top of your head to the front of your ear on both sides and clip one section out of the way with the crocodile clip.

2. Bring the free section of hair around the back of your head and pin it securely with a conventional bobby pin behind your ear. You may need two pins depending on the thickness of your hair. These pins will be hidden once you have completed the next step.

3. Release the clipped section and bring that around the back of your head, on top of the other section, to the other side of your head. Pin securely by inserting a gold metallic bobby pin vertically from the bottom of the hair up.

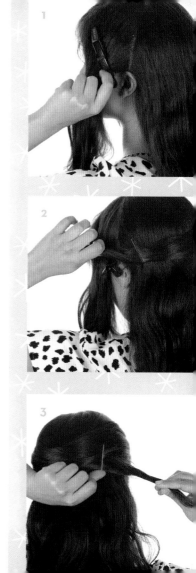

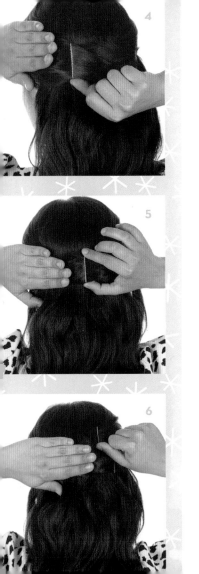

4. Insert a gold glitter pin in the same vertical manner on the opposite side of your head. These two pins will be the starting point of two large stars.

5. Insert a gold metallic pin in the same vertical manner at the back of your head. This will secure your hair even more and begin the third star.

6. Insert a mini gold glitter pin vertically above and between the gold metallic pins. Now the base for all four stars is complete. You've finished the hard part! The rest of the steps explain how to finish one star.

7. Choose one of your secured pins and insert a matching pin across the vertical pin but at an angle. If it looks like a lopsided plus sign, you did it right!

8. Insert a matching pin across those two pins in the opposite direction, so you end up with a six-pointed star.

9. Repeat steps 7 through 9 for the other vertical pins to create three more stars.

STYLE TIPS

Once the pins are in place, you can move them around slightly to get the star shape you desire.

If your hair doesn't feel totally secure by the end, insert a few more conventional bobby pins to match your hair color where you need them.

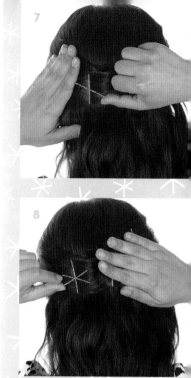

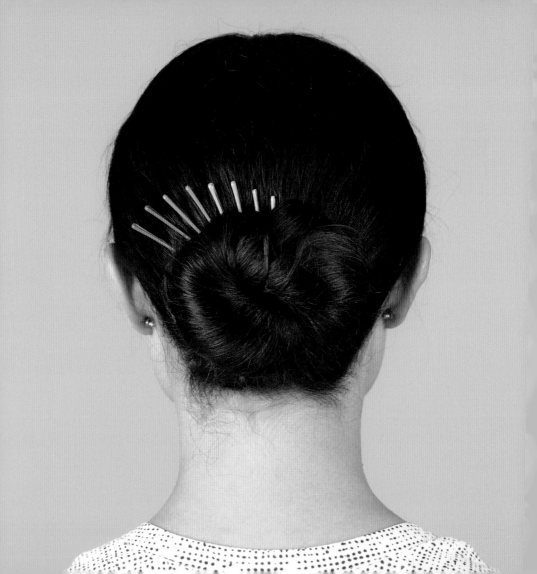

OMBRÉ FAN

Pink ombré pins adorn a sleek bun with a touch of fun,
suitable for your classiest event.

DIFFICULTY LEVEL

easy

IDEAL HAIR LENGTH

*shoulder
and longer*

MATERIALS

boar-bristle brush

hair elastic

conventional bobby pins to match
your hair color

2 sets of ombré bobby pins in any
color (at least 4 to a set)

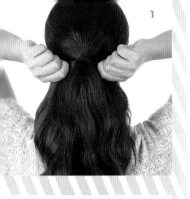

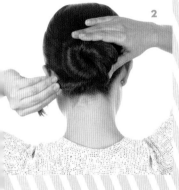

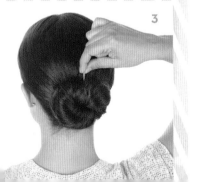

1. Using the boar-bristle brush, smooth and gather your hair into a low ponytail, then secure with a hair elastic.

2. Create a bun and secure with conventional bobby pins to match your hair color as needed.

3. Once the bun is secure, insert your lightest-colored pin vertically with the open side facing down into the top and center of the bun. Push it down so about a third of the pin is showing.

4. Insert the same color pin to the left of the first pin, pushing it down toward the center of the bun. Do not push this pin down as far into the bun; it should stick up slightly higher than the first pin.

5. Insert the slightly darker pin in ombré order to the left of the second pin in the same manner. This pin should be slightly higher than the second pin.

6. Continue inserting pins around the bun. Always insert two of the same shade and then move on to the next darker shade, so that the last pin you insert is the darkest. Each pin should sit a little higher in the bun. Voilà! Now you have a pretty, colorful "fan" to decorate your bun.

STYLE TIPS

To master this look it is important that all the pins have the same amount of space between them.

If you need help creating a bun, here's how to do it: Take the hair in your low ponytail and twist it. Then twist your hair around the hair elastic and around itself to create the bun. Stick the ends of your hair under the bun and secure the entire thing with conventional bobby pins.

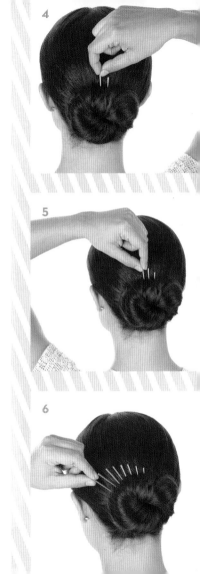

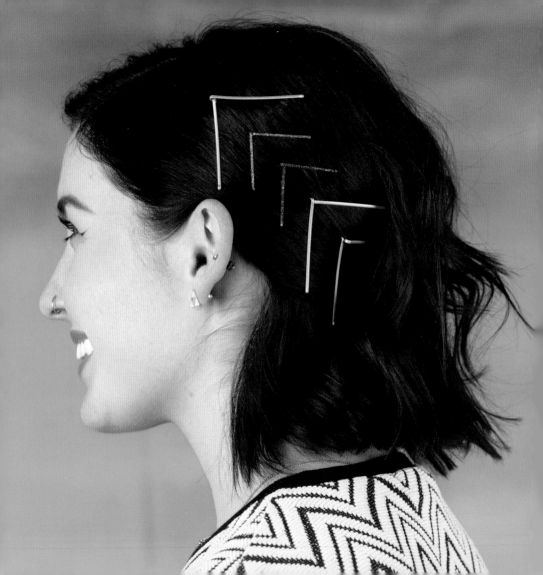

SIDE-SWEPT CHEVRON

A faux-shaved style for your inner wild child.

DIFFICULTY LEVEL

easy

IDEAL HAIR LENGTH

chin and longer

MATERIALS

fine-toothed comb

boar-bristle brush

conventional bobby pins to match your hair color

6 silver bobby pins

2 mini teal glitter bobby pins

2 mini blue glitter bobby pins

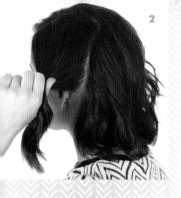

1. Using your fine-toothed comb, create a deep side part.

2. Grab a section of hair from the parted side that extends from the crown of your head to the back of your ear.

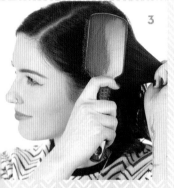

3. Using a boar-bristle brush, smooth this section of hair.

4. Pull this section of hair tightly around your head and under the rest of your hair. Pin it in place using a conventional bobby pin or two.

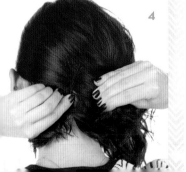

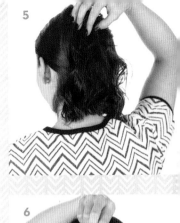

5. Use your hand to tousle your hair over this pinned section. The pins will now be obscured by your hair.

6. Insert a silver bobby pin, angling down and back into the tight side of your hair just above your ear.

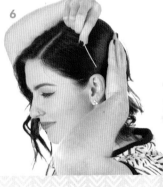

7. Starting from the same place, insert another silver pin, angling up and back to create an inverted V shape.

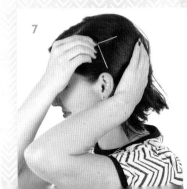

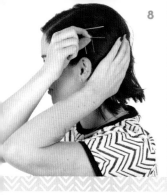

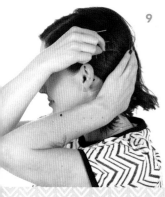

8. About ½ in/12 mm below this inverted V, insert two mini teal glitter pins in the same manner.

9. About ½ in/12 mm below the teal pins, insert mini blue glitter pins in the same manner.

10. Finish with two more rows of silver pins, leaving ½ in/12 mm between the V's.

STYLE TIPS

To master this look, it is important for all of the pins to have the same amount of space between them.

Use your boar-bristle brush to get your hair super smooth and tight to your head on the one side to really drive home that faux-shaved look. Mist with hair spray before you start pinning so it stays super sleek and in place.

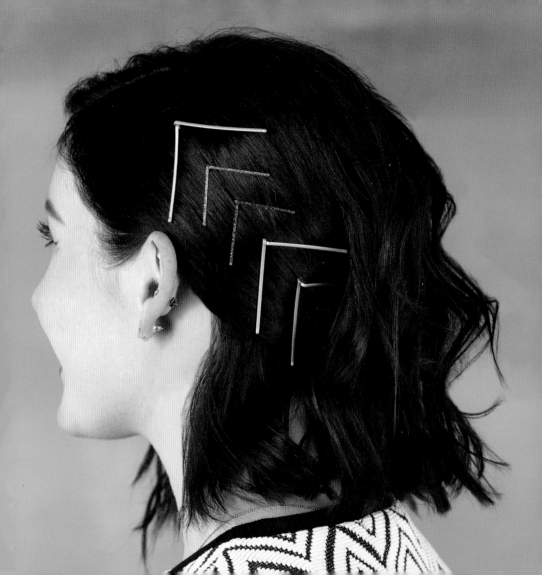

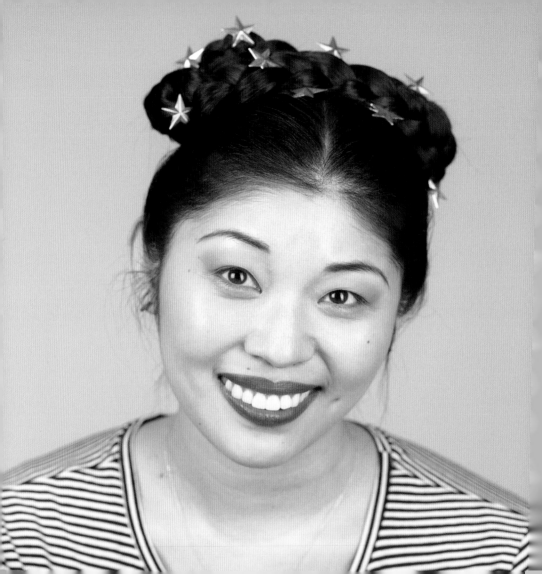

CONSTELLATION BRAID CROWN

Make your hair a statement piece with this star-studded braided look.

hard

midback and longer

MATERIALS

fine-toothed comb

2 hair elastics

2 clear hair elastics

conventional bobby pins to match your hair color

10 or more gold and silver star-tipped bobby pins

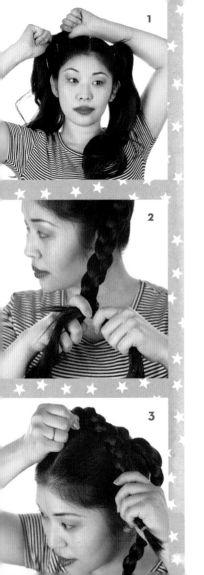

1. Using the comb, part your hair in the center and create two high pigtails. Secure with elastics.

2. Create a simple braid out of each pigtail: Divide one pigtail into three sections and cross the right section over the middle section. Then cross the left section over the middle section. Continue crossing "right over middle" and "left over middle" until the braid is complete. Secure with a clear elastic. Repeat with the other pigtail.

3. Pull your right braid across the top of your head and secure it in place with conventional bobby pins.

4. Continue pulling that braid over and wrap it behind the hair elastic of the left pigtail braid. Secure behind the elastic with conventional bobby pins.

5. Take your left braid and pull it across the top of your head and behind the first braid. Secure everything well with conventional bobby pins.

6. Insert gold and silver star-tipped bobby pins throughout the braid crown at various angles, some against your head and others peeking out from behind the crown. Try to hide the pin itself within the braid so that just the star is showing.

STYLE TIPS

Spray your hair with hair spray as you are braiding to achieve a sleek braid with no fly-aways.

The length of your hair will determine how much wrapping you do with your braids. No matter what, make sure you tuck the ends of your braids into the center of the braid crown so the elastics are hidden.

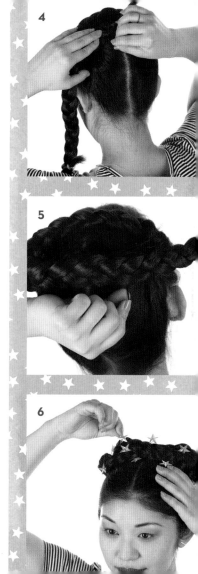

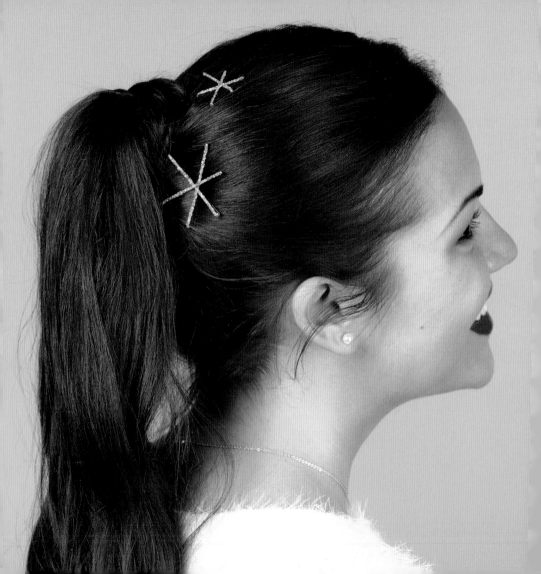

VINTAGE PONYTAIL

Starbursts take this polished pony all the way back to the 1960s for a vintage look that's both playful and glamorous.

DIFFICULTY LEVEL

medium

IDEAL HAIR LENGTH

shoulder and longer

MATERIALS

fine-toothed comb

2 crocodile clips

boar-bristle brush

hair elastic

conventional bobby pins to match your hair color

3 silver glitter bobby pins

6 mini silver glitter bobby pins

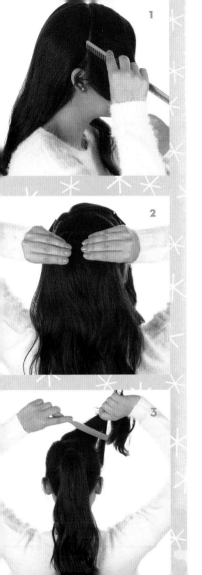

1. Using the comb, create a side part. Then create two sections of hair by moving the comb from the part to the top of one ear, then repeating on the other side. Clip the hair on both sides out of the way with the crocodile clips.

2. Using the boar-bristle brush to smooth the hair, pull the rest of your hair into a high ponytail and secure with an elastic.

3. Release one of the front sections of hair and tease lightly with the brush to create a little volume.

4. Pull the teased section loosely back to your ponytail and swoop the hair under your elastic.

5. Twist the hair around the elastic until it is completely covered. Secure the ends into the ponytail with a conventional bobby pin and hide it underneath the ponytail.

6. Repeat steps 3 through 5 on the other side.

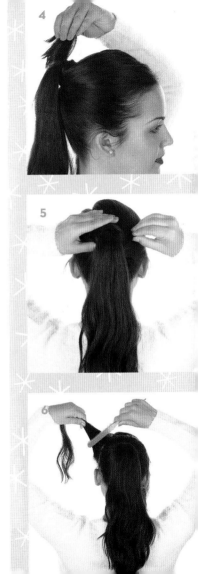

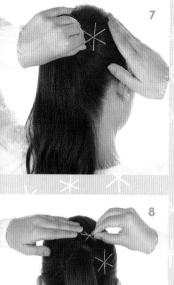

7. Insert silver glitter pins in a starburst formation (see Starburst Crown, page 27) to the right of your ponytail.

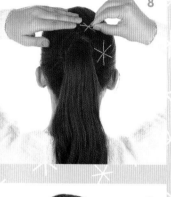

8. Insert mini silver glitter pins in a starburst formation above and slightly to the right of your ponytail.

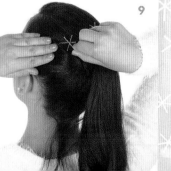

9. Insert mini silver glitter pins in a starburst formation to the left of your ponytail.

STYLE TIPS

Use a curling iron to curl the end of your ponytail, and mist with hair spray to help the curl hold.

When teasing the front sections of your hair, lightly mist them with hair spray or texturizing spray, and brush them into place with a boar-bristle brush before wrapping them around the ponytail and pinning them into place. This will help the hair hold together.

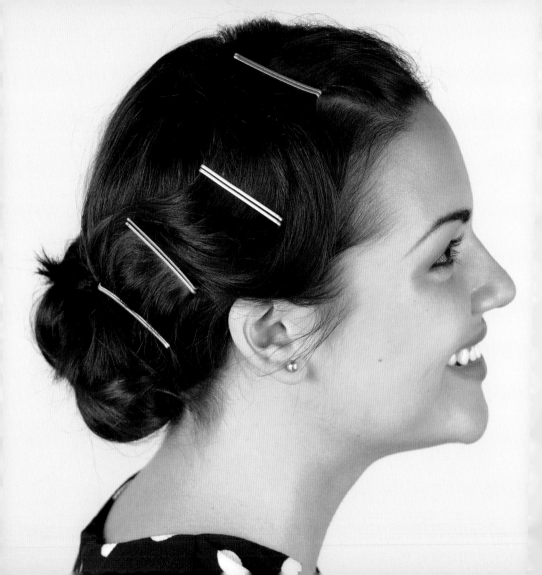

FAUX FINGER WAVE

Channel your inner Zelda Fitzgerald because
tonight you're gonna party like it's 1929.

DIFFICULTY LEVEL

hard

IDEAL HAIR LENGTH

*chin and
longer*

MATERIALS

fine-toothed comb

curling iron or curling wand

boar-bristle brush

8 gold metallic bobby pins

8 silver metallic bobby pins

1 hair elastic

conventional bobby pins to match
your hair color

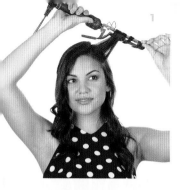

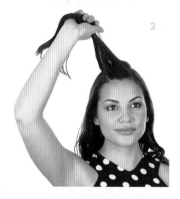

1. Using the comb, part your hair on one side. Using a curling iron, loosely curl all your hair.

2. Grab a 4-in/10-cm section of hair from your hairline back along your part. You will be working with this section of hair through step 7.

3. Using the boar-bristle brush, smooth this section of hair forward.

4. Sweep the section back and insert two gold bobby pins, angling up and away from your face, about 3 in/7.5 cm back from your hairline.

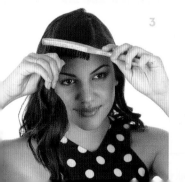

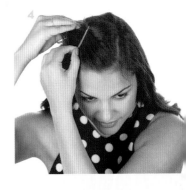

5. Hold the section of hair behind the gold pins and push it forward. This should create an S shape. Insert two silver bobby pins in the center of the curve, this time pointing the pins toward your face. If your hair is thick, the bobby pin probably won't cover the hair all the way. Don't worry about it! The next pin will keep the S swoop in place.

6. Now push the section of hair behind the silver bobby pins and create an S curve going in the opposite direction. Insert two gold pins in the center of that curve, this time pointing the pins up and away from your face.

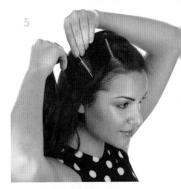

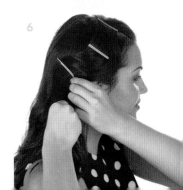

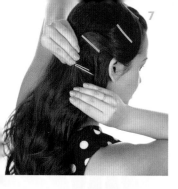

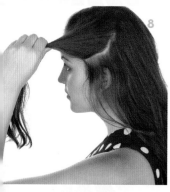

7. Once again push that section of hair forward and insert two silver pins in the center of the curve, pointing the pins toward your face, just like in step 5.

8. Grab a 4-in/10-cm section on the opposite side of your head. Repeat steps 3 through 7 on this section of hair.

9. Once you finish pinning both sides, gather your hair into a low ponytail and secure with an elastic.

10. Finish by creating a bun and securing it with bobby pins to match your hair.

STYLE TIPS

If you need help creating a bun, check out the Ombré Fan (page 33).

If you have very short hair, skip the bun and either gather the remaining hair into a ponytail or leave it free.

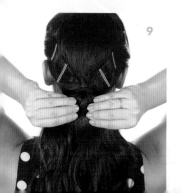

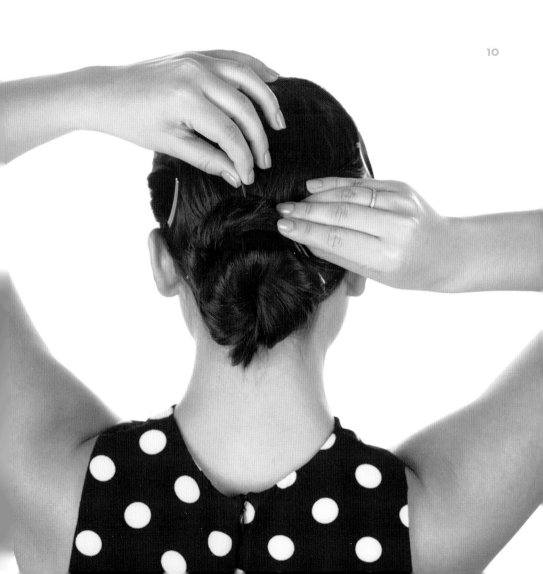

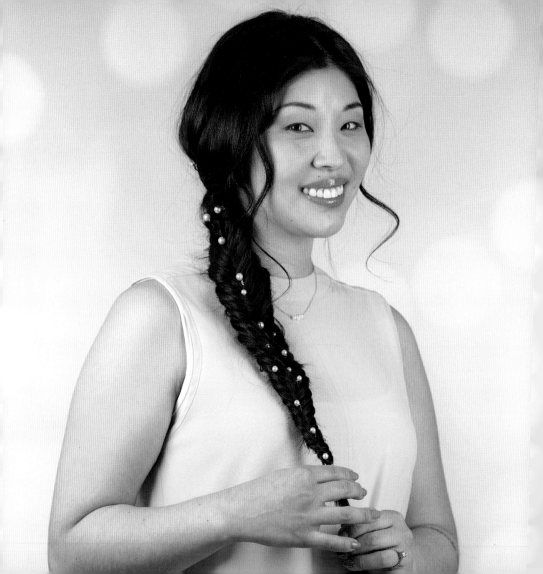

MERMAID BRAID

This loose romantic braid dotted with white pearls is just too elegant to stay under the sea.

DIFFICULTY LEVEL

easy to medium

IDEAL HAIR LENGTH

midback and longer

MATERIALS

texturizing spray

curling iron

clear hair elastic

pearl-tipped bobby pins, enough to place down your braid

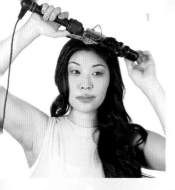

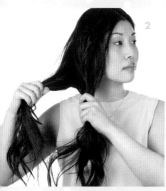

1. Mist your hair lightly all over with texturizing spray. Then curl your hair quickly to create loose curls all over.

2. Sweep all of your hair over to one side and divide into two equal sections.

3. Create a fishtail braid by bringing a small piece of hair from the left section over and into the right section.

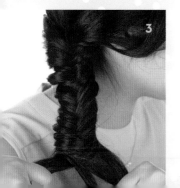

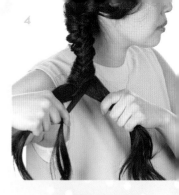

4. Next take a small piece from the right section over and into the left section.

5. Every time you cross a piece of hair over, pull both sections to make the braid tight.

6. Repeat steps 3 and 4 until the braid is finished.

7. Pinch the braid on either side and pull the braid apart gently so it becomes wider and slightly messy.

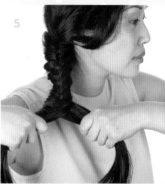

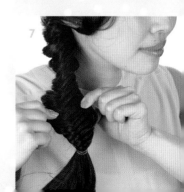

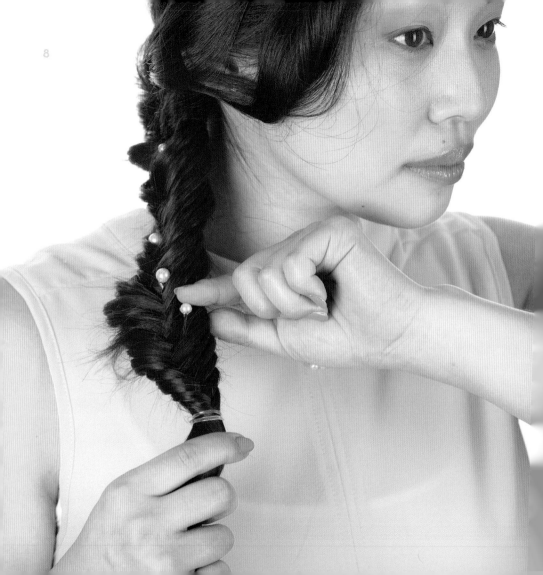

8. Take your pearl-tipped bobby pins and stick them, in a random arrangement, into your braid vertically so the pins disappear but you can see the pearls.

STYLE TIPS

Pull forward some pieces of hair from around your face and curl them to get an even more relaxed mermaid look.

If your hair is layered, you may end up with a lot of hair sticking out of your braid. To help combat this problem, mist your hair lightly with hair spray once you have it in two sections, but before you start your braid. Then, when the braid is done, spray it again with hair spray and let it completely dry before lightly pulling your braid apart.

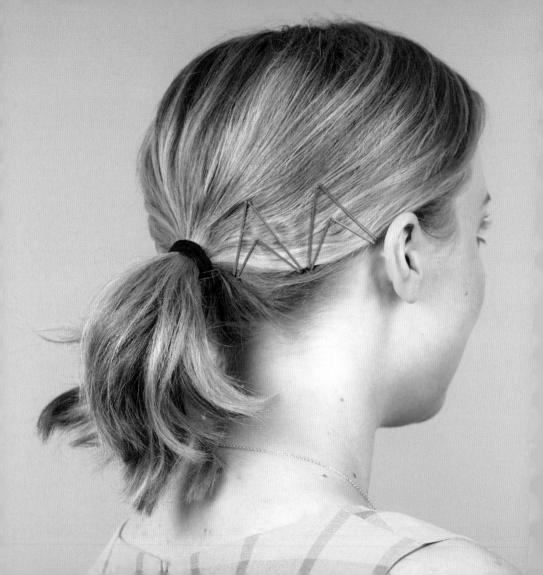

GALACTIC LOW PONY

Orange pins dress up a casual ponytail for an on-the-go look that's out of this world. Match your nails to your pins for a truly space-age style.

MATERIALS

fine-toothed comb

1 hair elastic

4 orange bobby pins

4 mini orange bobby pins

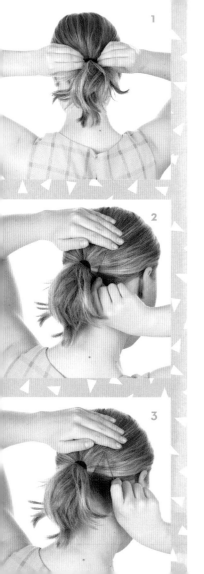

1. Use the comb to part your hair at your desired location—center or side—and gather into a low ponytail. Secure with an elastic.

2. Using two standard orange pins, create an upside-down V shape to the left of your ponytail. To do this, insert one bobby pin up and angled to the right and then insert another pin about 1½ in/4 cm from the first pin and angle it up and to the left.

3. The ends of each pin should meet in the center.

4. Starting from the bottom of the first bobby pin, insert a mini orange bobby pin going up and toward the center of the V.

5. Starting from the bottom of the second pin, insert another mini orange bobby pin going up and toward the center of the V. Once this step is complete you should have one inverted V with a smaller inverted V inside it.

6. Repeat steps 2 through 4 just to the right of your first V.

STYLE TIPS

I prefer a certain amount of asymmetry in style, but if you're a symmetry person, don't hesitate to create this pin design on both sides of your ponytail.

This is a perfect style for my super-short-haired people! I think it looks best with a small ponytail, and the pins help hold pesky short pieces in place. Use a light mist of hair spray when brushing your hair into your ponytail to help hold it in place.

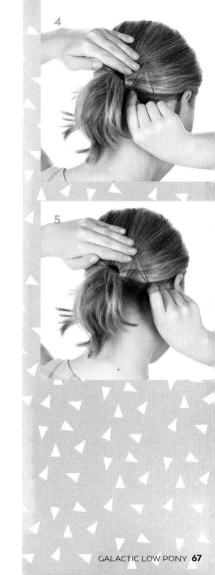

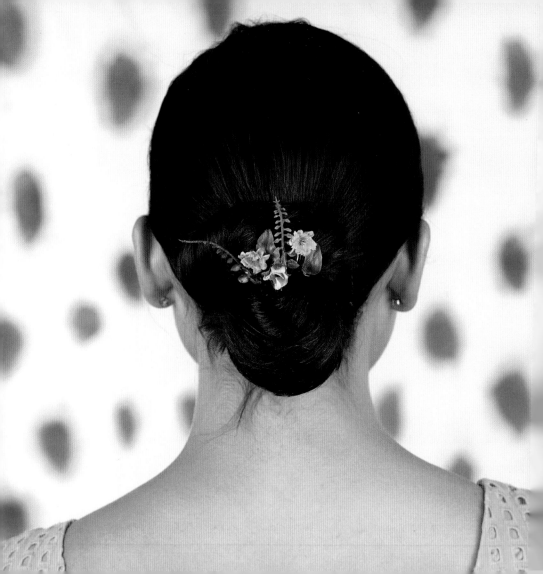

FLOWER BOUQUET

You'll be the belle of the garden party with this bouquet
of tiny silk flowers tucked in your hair.

DIFFICULTY LEVEL

easy

IDEAL HAIR LENGTH

chin and longer

MATERIALS

fine-toothed comb

1 hair elastic

conventional bobby pins to match
your hair color

3 or 4 flower-tipped bobby pins

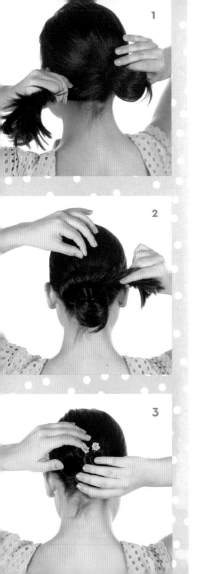

1. Use the comb to part your hair at your desired location (center or side) and pull it into a mid-low ponytail. When you are looping your hair elastic for the last time, do not pull the hair all the way through. Instead leave your hair in a small vertical loop.

2. Twist the loose hair that you did not pull through and wrap it around the elastic holding your looped hair. Insert conventional bobby pins into the center of the ponytail, from the top down, to keep the twist in place. Use as many pins as you need for the twisted hair to feel secure.

3. Insert a few flower-tipped bobby pins into the top of your loop so it looks like the flowers are coming out of the loop.

STYLE TIPS

If you have very short hair, you probably won't have any leftover length to wrap around the loop. Don't worry! Simply leave the leftover hair you didn't pull through where it is at the side of your hair elastic.

To create more visual interest, insert your flower-tipped bobby pins at varying heights. Think of it like a real bouquet.

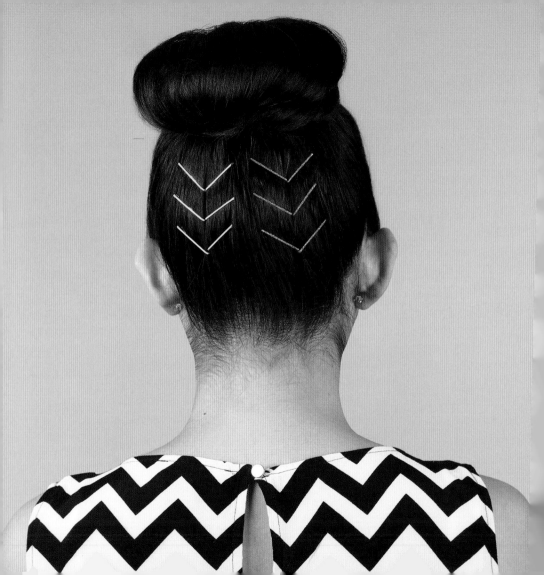

SKY-HIGH BUN

Colorful chevron pins create a graphic statement on this sleek bun. Pair it with a leather jacket or all-black ensemble to take the look over the edge.

easy to medium

shoulder and longer

MATERIALS

1 hair elastic

boar-bristle brush

conventional bobby pins to match your hair color

6 mini yellow glitter bobby pins

6 mini teal glitter bobby pins

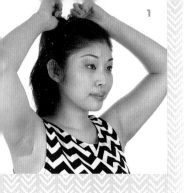

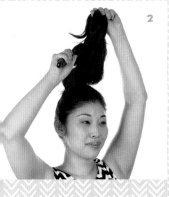

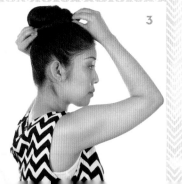

1. Gather your hair into a very high ponytail. (Sometimes it helps if you flip your head upside down to do this!) Secure with an elastic.

2. Grab the ends of your ponytail and hold them straight up in the air. Tease your ponytail by brushing the hair from the ends toward your head with a boar-bristle brush.

3. Take your now-very-messy ponytail and twirl it around the hair elastic to form a bun. Secure it in place with conventional bobby pins.

4. Starting near your neck on the left side of your head, insert two mini yellow glitter pins so they create a wide V shape. Insert the first pin angling up and to the left, and the second pin angling up and to the right.

5. Create two more yellow V's directly above the first one. The V's should be about 1 in/2.5 cm to 1½ in/4 cm apart, depending on how much room you have below your bun.

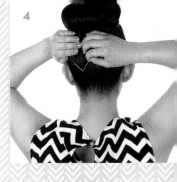

6. Now switch to the right side and repeat steps 4 and 5, this time using mini teal glitter pins.

STYLE TIPS

If you want your ponytail to be super tight and sleek against your head, wet your hair slightly at the roots and use a boar-bristle brush to smooth your hair into place before securing.

If you need help creating a bun, check out Ombré Fan (page 33).

Pair this style with a chevron or color-blocked shirt for an overall graphic look.

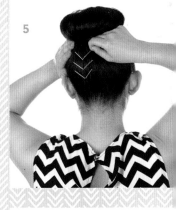

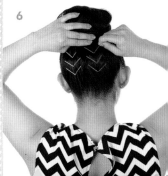

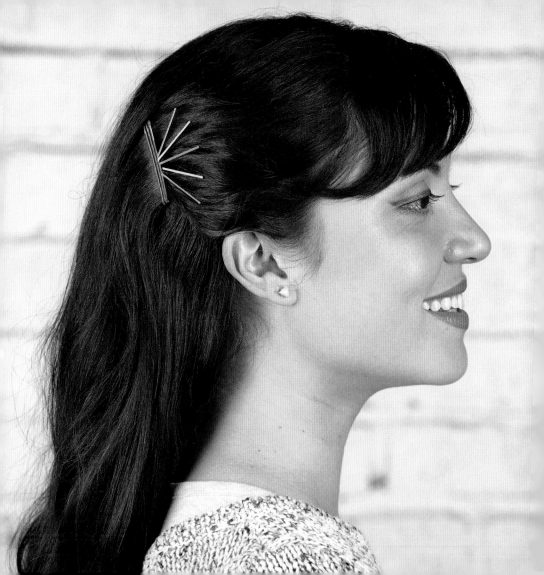

SETTING SUN

This look features rays of orange and yellow pins that will light up your hair so you can light up the room.

DIFFICULTY LEVEL

medium

IDEAL HAIR LENGTH

chin and longer

MATERIALS

curling iron

fine-toothed comb

3 dark orange bobby pins

3 mini light orange bobby pins

2 mini yellow bobby pins

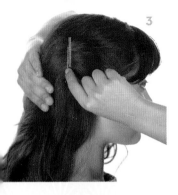

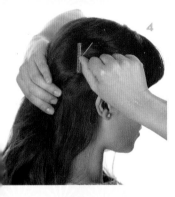

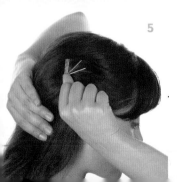

1. Using the curling iron, curl your hair quickly to create loose curls all over.

2. With your fine-toothed comb, create a side part.

3. On one side of your head, grab a 4-in/10-cm section from your part to above your ear, gently pull it away from your face, and secure with three dark orange bobby pins placed flush against each other.

4. Starting from the vertical center of the pin closest to your face, insert a mini light orange pin, angling it up and out on a diagonal.

5. Starting from the vertical center once again, insert a mini yellow pin, angling it up and out at slightly less of an angle.

6. Again from the vertical center, insert a mini light orange pin straight out at a 90-degree angle so it is perpendicular to the vertical pins.

7. Beginning again from the center, insert a mini yellow pin, angling it down and out on a diagonal.

8. Last, insert a mini light orange pin from the vertical center, angling it down and out at an even greater angle.

STYLE TIPS

Don't have time to curl your hair? No problem! This style looks great on any hair texture.

Depending on the thickness of your hair, you can play around with step 3. If your hair is thin, perhaps you only need two pins. Conversely, if your hair is thick, add as many pins as you need for your hair to feel secure.

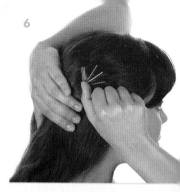

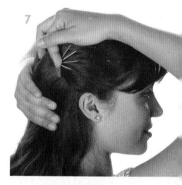

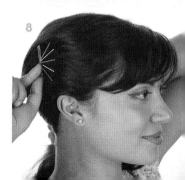

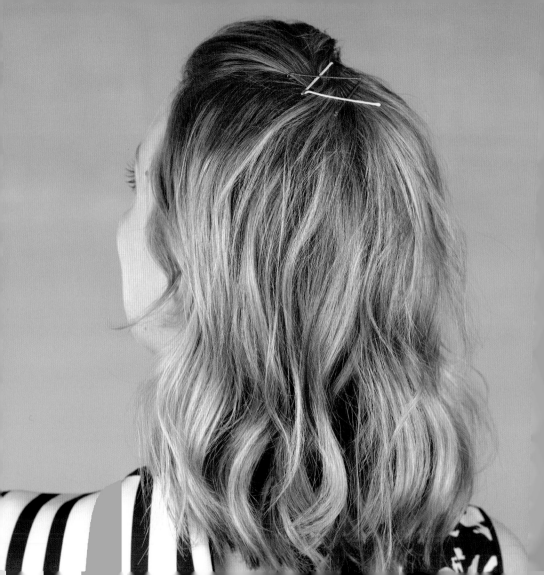

X MARKS THE SPOT

This simple style is perfect for keeping hair out of your face while you take on the day.

DIFFICULTY LEVEL

easy

IDEAL HAIR LENGTH

chin and longer

MATERIALS

hair spray or texturizing spray

2 yellow bobby pins

2 pink bobby pins

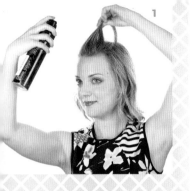

1. Grab a 3-in/7.5-cm-wide section of hair from above your forehead and mist lightly with hair spray or texturizing spray so the hair will hold once pinned.

2. Twist the hair once or twice.

3. Secure the section to the top of your head by inserting one yellow bobby pin diagonally across the section.

4. On the opposite side of the section, insert one pink pin diagonally and across the yellow pin, creating a shallow X shape.

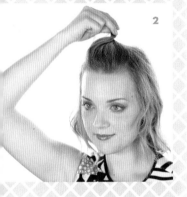

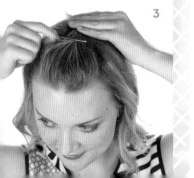

5. Switching back to the first side, insert a second pink pin at the tip of the first pink pin. Angle it away from your face in the same direction as the yellow pin.

6. On the opposite side, insert a second yellow pin at the tip of the first yellow pin, creating a second shallow X shape directly behind the first.

STYLE TIPS

For the full effect, make sure the ends of your pink pins touch, and the ends of your yellow pins touch, to make two overlapping V's.

This is a great go-to style if you're trying to grow out some pesky bangs!

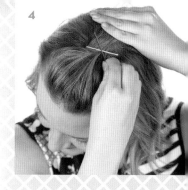

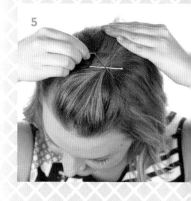

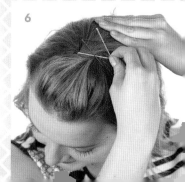

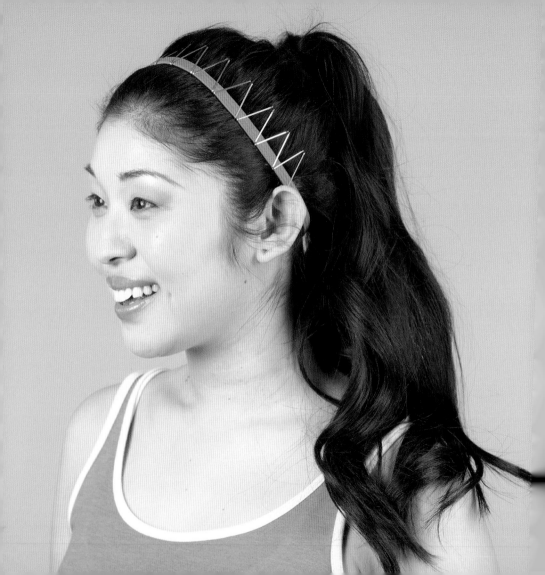

SPORTY

Spice up a simple headband with mini gold pins for an unbeatable look that will take you over the finish line.

DIFFICULTY LEVEL

easy

IDEAL HAIR LENGTH

shoulder and longer

MATERIALS

hair elastic

thin sports headband

15 to 20 mini gold bobby pins

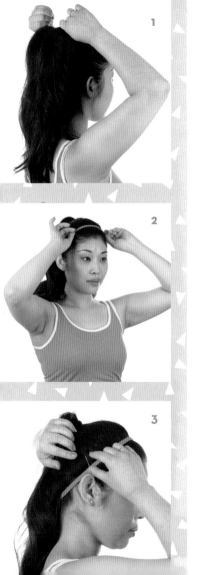

1. Pull your hair into a high ponytail and secure with an elastic.

2. Wrap the sports headband around your head, about 1½ in/4 cm back from your hairline.

3. Starting from above your ear, insert a mini gold bobby pin across the headband on a slight upward diagonal.

4. Now insert a mini bobby pin about an inch above that on a slight downward diagonal so that the tips of the two bobby pins meet.

5. Repeat step 3 and 4 over and over, making sure all opposite ends of the bobby pins touch. A zigzag pattern will start to emerge. Continue pinning until you get to the top of your other ear.

STYLE TIPS

Before you create your ponytail, put your sports headband over your head and let it hang around your neck until you're ready to put it on. This way you won't mess up your ponytail while getting the headband over your head.

If your ponytail is super long and you need your hair further secured away from your face, gather your ponytail into a braid or a bun. Or a braided bun!

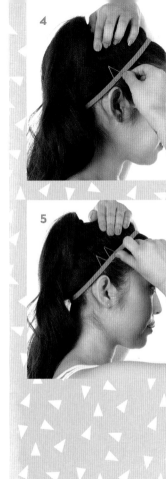

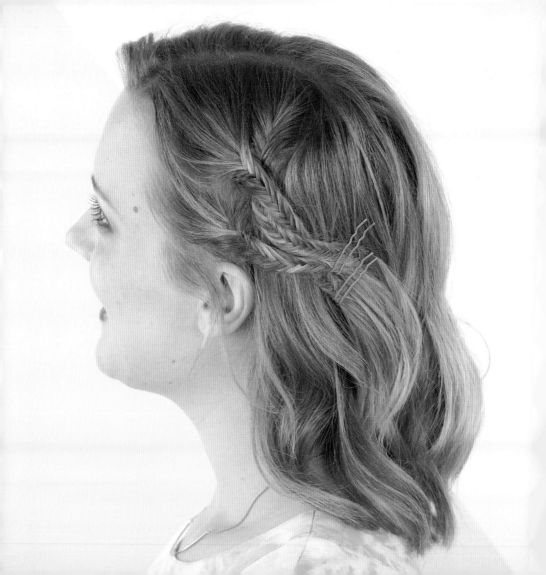

TRIPLE BRAIDS

Three fishtail braids and bright glitter pins create a beautiful focal point for this soft and loose style.

MATERIALS

fine-toothed comb

curling iron

3 clear hair elastics

4 mini blue glitter bobby pins

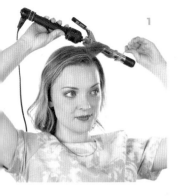

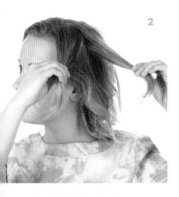

1. Using the comb, part your hair on one side. Then use the curling iron to create loose waves all over.

2. On the same side as your part, grab two 3-in/7.5-cm sections of hair. They don't necessarily need to be even, as this look should have a loose style.

3. Braid each of these two sections into a fishtail braid, secure each with a small clear elastic, and lightly pull the braids apart to widen. (See Mermaid Braid, page 59.)

4. Take another 3-in/7.5-cm section of hair below the first braid and create another fishtail braid.

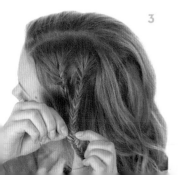

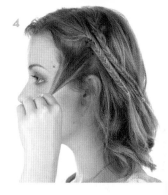

5. Now that you have three braids, take the first braid and cross it over the top of the second.

6. Cross the same two braids again so the second braid is now on top. Let the first braid drop down and don't worry about it for now.

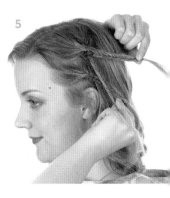

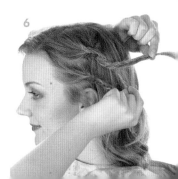

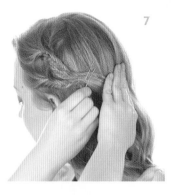

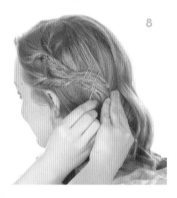

7. Pull the third braid back and join it under the second braid. Secure both the second and third braids by inserting two blue glitter pins up and on a diagonal.

8. Now take the end of the first braid, pull it back and down, and secure with two more blue glitter pins so that they are securing the third braid as well as the first and second.

9. Remove all the hair elastics after the braids are in place.

STYLE TIPS

This is a perfect style for a short bob that has slightly longer hair in the front than in the back.

Don't have time to bang out three fishtails? Skip the third braid and just follow the steps for the first two braids.

FOURTH OF JULY

Make your hair sparkle with this fireworks display featuring two buns surrounded by glittering red, white, and blue pins.

DIFFICULTY LEVEL

easy to medium

IDEAL HAIR LENGTH

collar bone and longer

MATERIALS

fine-toothed comb

2 hair elastics

conventional bobby pins to match your hair color

6 mini white glitter bobby pins

4 mini blue glitter bobby pins

2 mini red glitter bobby pins

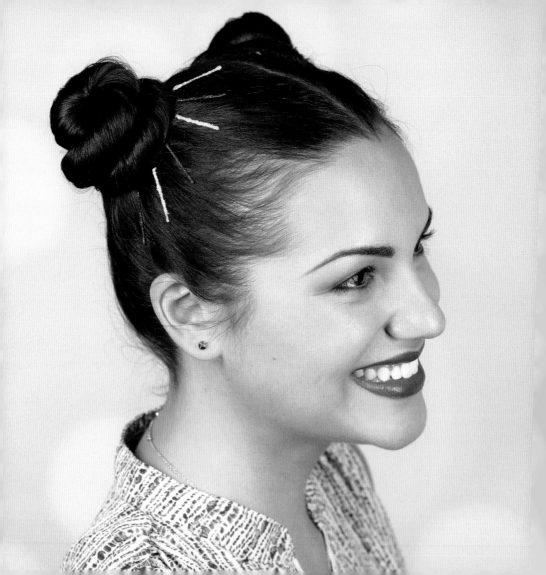

1. Using the comb, part your hair in the center. Gather your tresses into two high pigtails and secure with hair elastics.

2. Twist the pigtails into two buns and secure with conventional bobby pins.

3. Insert a mini white glitter pin at the interior base of one bun, angling it toward your part.

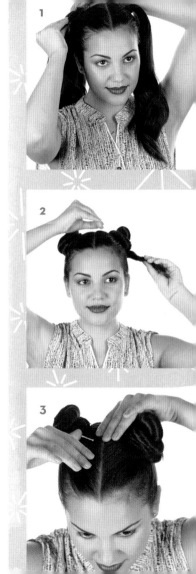

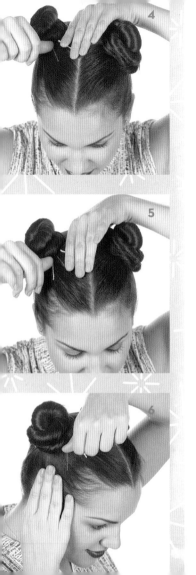

4. Next to it, insert a mini blue glitter pin, angling it slightly more toward your front hairline.

5. Next to your blue pin, insert another mini white glitter pin, angling it straight forward toward your hairline.

6. Then insert a mini red glitter pin, this one angled slightly down.

7. Insert one last mini white glitter pin, angling down toward the front of your ear.

8. Last, insert a mini blue glitter pin, angling it straight down toward your ear.

9. Repeat steps 3 through 8 on the other bun.

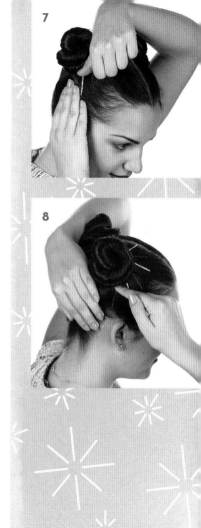

STYLE TIPS

Use a boar-bristle brush to get your hair super smooth against your head. This will help the sparkle pins really pop.

If your hair is too short to coil into buns, try this: When pulling your ponytail through the elastic for the final time, don't pull the hair all the way through; instead leave a loop, which will create a similar bun effect. (See Flower Bouquet, page 69.)

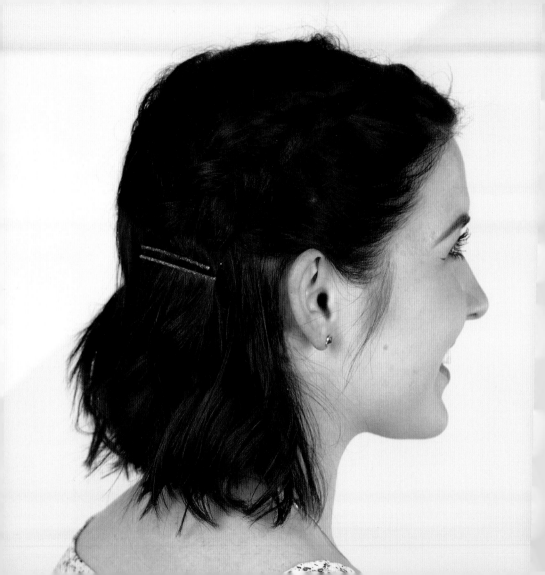

DOUBLE DUTCH BRAIDS

Double the fun with this braided style perfect for short-haired ladies. This casual look is an adorable way to keep the hair off your face on a hot summer day.

DIFFICULTY LEVEL

medium to hard

IDEAL HAIR LENGTH

chin and longer

MATERIALS

fine-toothed comb

texturizing spray or hair spray

4 green glitter bobby pins

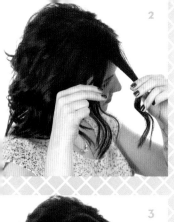

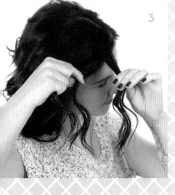

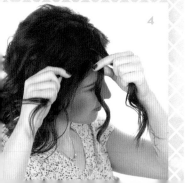

1. Using the comb, part your hair at your desired location and grab a small section of hair from the front of your head on one side.

2. Split that section into three equal pieces to begin your side Dutch braid.

3. Take the right piece and cross it under the middle piece.

4. Next take the left piece and cross it under the middle piece (which is actually your right piece).

5. Then cross the right piece under the middle piece, but this time add in some hair from the right-hand side.

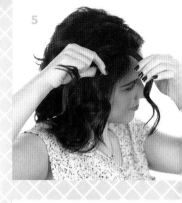

6. Cross the left side under the middle, this time adding some hair from the left-hand side.

7. Continue the braid down the side of your head until you get behind your ear. Here, insert one green glitter pin away from your ear.

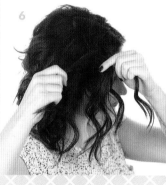

8. Insert a second green glitter pin facing toward your ear to secure the braid.

9. Repeat all steps on the second side.

STYLE TIPS

Lightly spray short hair with hair spray or texturizing spray before you start braiding to help hold short hairs in the braid.

To mix up the look, braid all the way down your head and gather the unbraided hair into a small, low ponytail.

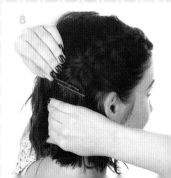

FISHTAIL WRAP

Yellow glitter pins accent two sweet braids in this style perfect for long-haired gals. Match your nails to the pins for an extra pop of yellow.

DIFFICULTY LEVEL

medium

IDEAL HAIR LENGTH

midback and longer

MATERIALS

fine-toothed comb

2 hair elastics

2 clear hair elastics

conventional bobby pins to match your hair color

15 or more mini yellow glitter bobby pins

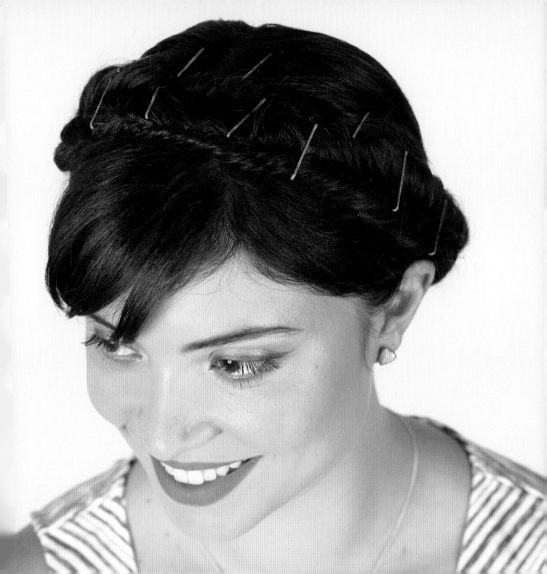

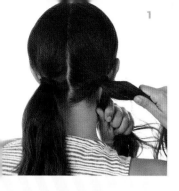

1. Using the comb, part your hair down the center and gather into two low pigtails at the back of your head. Secure with hair elastics.

2. Make a fishtail braid out of each pigtail. (See Mermaid Braid, page 59.) Secure the ends of the braids with clear elastics.

3. Take one braid, wrap it across your head toward the opposite ear, and secure with as many conventional bobby pins as you need.

4. Wrap the other section across your head toward the other ear and secure with more conventional bobby pins.

5. Insert mini yellow glitter pins at random throughout the braids facing straight back.

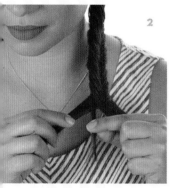

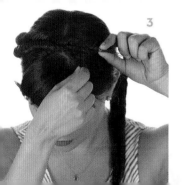

STYLE TIPS

Fishtail braids work best on hair that is all one length or doesn't have a lot of layering. Heavily layered hair tends to pop out of this braid easily.

Create your pigtails at the back of your head, instead of right behind your ears. This will prevent the hair elastic from sticking out from your ears when you wrap the braids over your head.

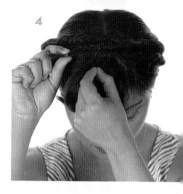

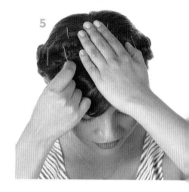

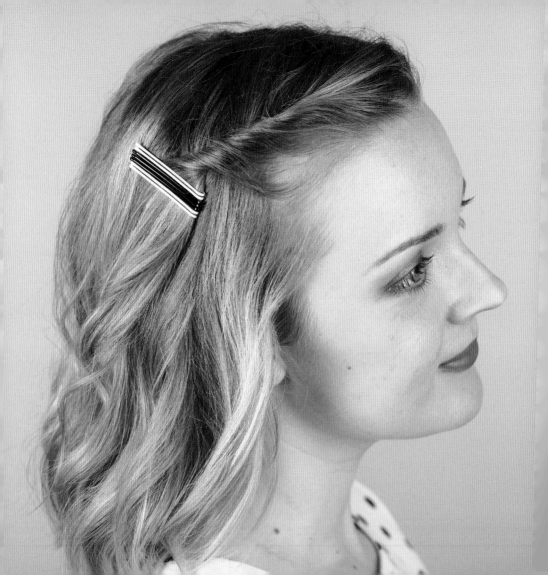

BLACK AND WHITE

A functional-yet-bold look for a casual hair day.

DIFFICULTY LEVEL

easy

IDEAL HAIR LENGTH

chin and longer

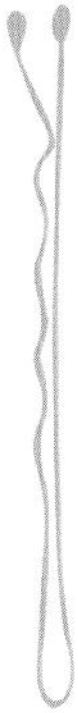

MATERIALS

curling iron

4 white bobby pins

3 black bobby pins

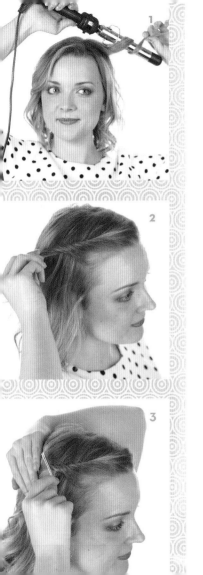

1. Put a loose wave in your hair all over by wrapping 2-in/5-cm sections around the curling iron and curling away from your face.

2. Grab a small section of hair at the front of your head and twist it back away from your face.

3. Insert two white bobby pins flush next to each other at the end of the twist to secure it.

4. Insert three black bobby pins flush against the white pins.

5. Insert two more white bobby pins flush against the black pins.

STYLE TIPS

This is a perfect style if you're growing out bangs.

If you have very dark hair, try swapping out the black bobby pins for a bright color that will pop against your hair.

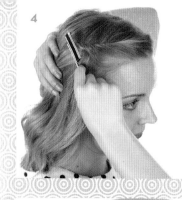

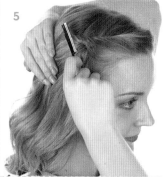

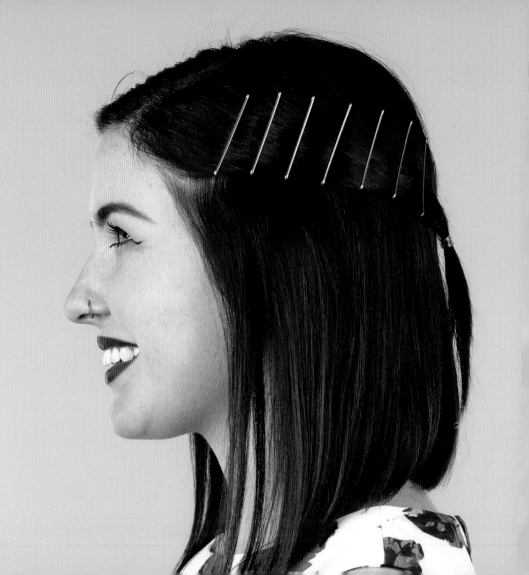

RENAISSANCE CROWN

Create a striking crown with simple pins that contrast with your hair for a look that's fit for a queen.

easy

shoulder and longer

MATERIALS

fine-toothed comb

flat iron

small clear hair elastic

conventional bobby pins to contrast with your hair color

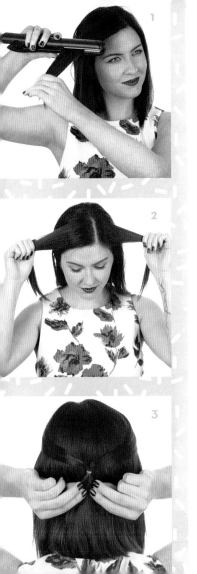

1. With your comb, create a side or center part. Smooth out your hair by taking small sections and running your flat iron down them from the roots to the tips.

2. Grab two small sections of hair from the front of your head on either side of your part.

3. Join these sections around the back of your head and secure with a small clear elastic.

4. Starting near your temple, insert a bobby pin into the pulled section of your hair, angled up and slightly back.

5. Insert another pin in the exact same manner about an inch down from the first pin.

6. Continue inserting your pins until you reach the hair elastic.

7. Repeat steps 4 through 6 on the opposite side of your head.

STYLE TIPS

To enhance this look, insert your pins closer together and add more on each side.

If you have long hair, try braiding the section that hangs down from the hair elastic.

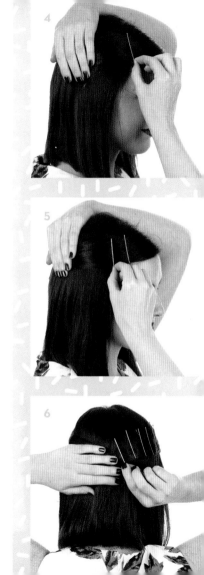

DECORATE YOUR PINS

You can find many different types of pins at beauty supply stores, but making your own pins is surprisingly quick and easy to do. The great thing about DIY pins is that you can make them exactly how you want. Match them to your outfit or makeup or nails—there are so many options! Everything you need to make your own pins can be found at any craft store. Or use items you already own, like jewelry you don't wear anymore. Here are a few quick projects for you to try out. Allow your imagination to run from there.

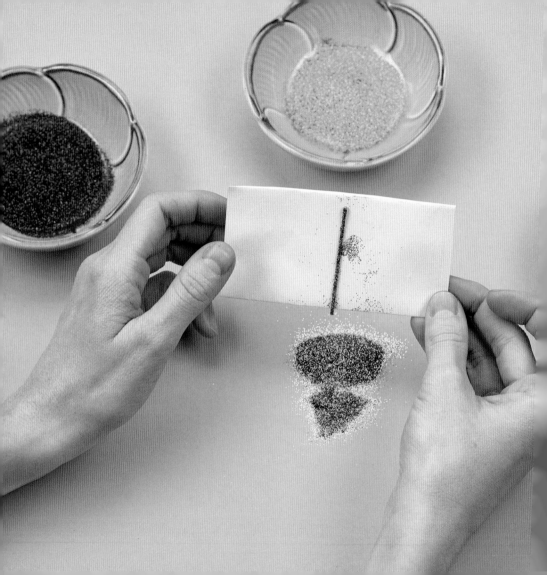

glitter pins

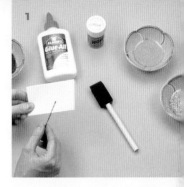

MATERIALS

conventional blond or brown bobby pins •
folded piece of paper or index card •
small strip of tinfoil • white glue •
sponge brush • extra-fine craft glitter

1. Clip a bobby pin onto a folded piece of paper.

2. Put some white glue onto a strip of foil and dip the tip of your sponge brush into the glue.

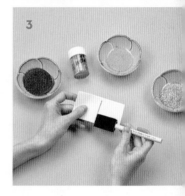

3. Press the glue onto the flat side of the bobby pin. Make sure that whole side is covered in glue.

4. Sprinkle glitter onto the glue-covered side of the pin until it is completely covered.

5. Lift the paper so the excess glitter falls away. Allow to dry.

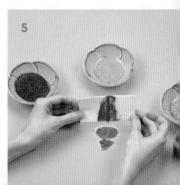

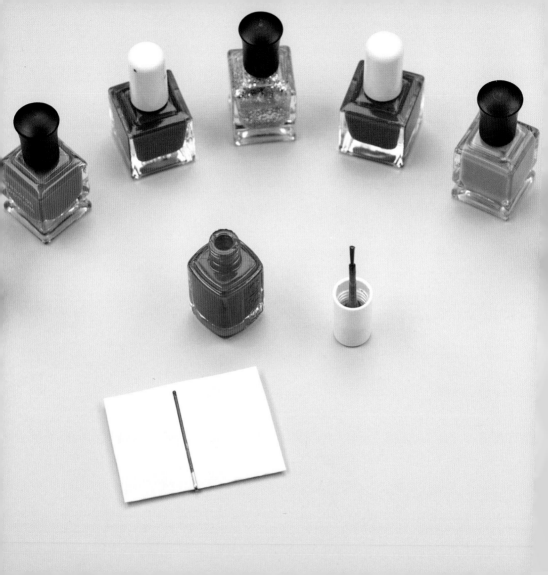

nail polish pins

conventional blond or white bobby pins •
folded piece of paper or index card •
nail polish in any color

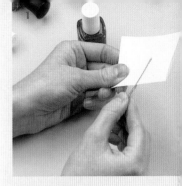

1. Clip a bobby pin onto the folded piece of paper so you can manipulate the pin without directly touching it.

2. Paint the flat side of your bobby pin with your nail polish brush. Allow to dry completely before using.

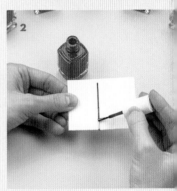

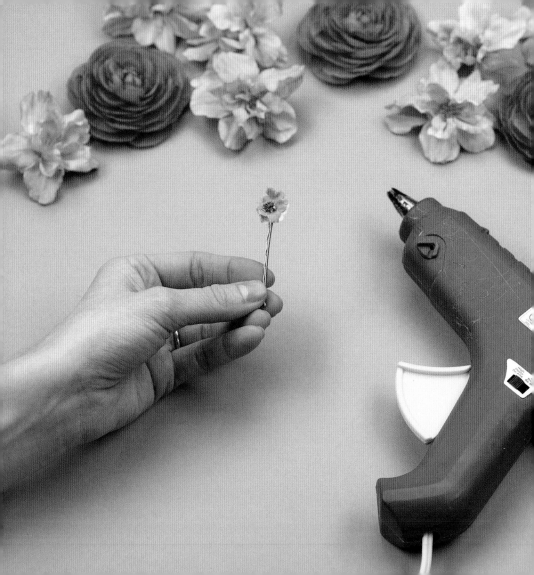

flower pins

MATERIALS

hot glue gun • small silk flowers • conventional bobby pins to match your hair color

1. Apply a generous dot of hot glue to the back of your silk flower.

2. Press the rounded end of the bobby pin into the hot glue and hold for a few seconds.

3. Apply another dot of hot glue on top of the pin, so the end of the bobby pin loop is entirely covered. Allow to dry completely before using.

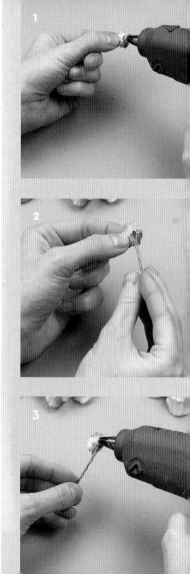

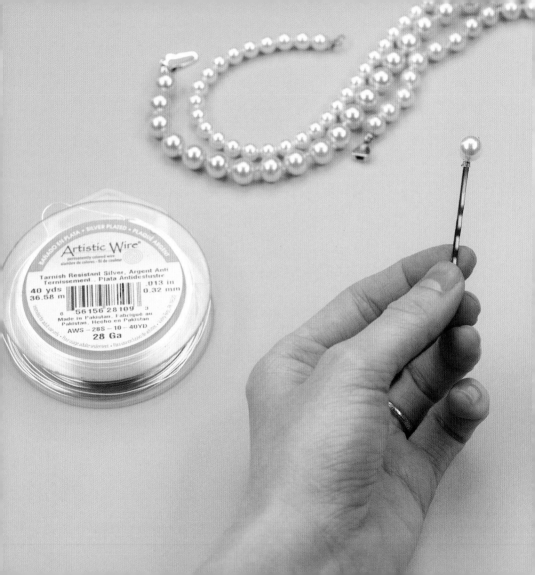

pearl pins

5 in/12 cm of 28-gauge jewelry wire •
conventional bobby pins to match your hair
color • craft scissors • pearl beads

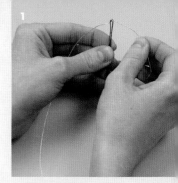

1. Insert the wire into the round end of the pin.
Loop the wire four or five times around the
loop of the bobby pin.

2. Using the scissors, clip one end of the wire
close to the pin.

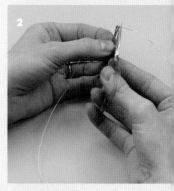

3. Insert the length of wire sticking out of the
other side of the pin through the pearl bead.

4. Pull the pearl tight against the loop of the
bobby pin and wrap the wire around the loop
of the pin 4 or 5 more times to secure the
pearl.

5. Clip the remaining length of wire.

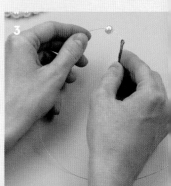

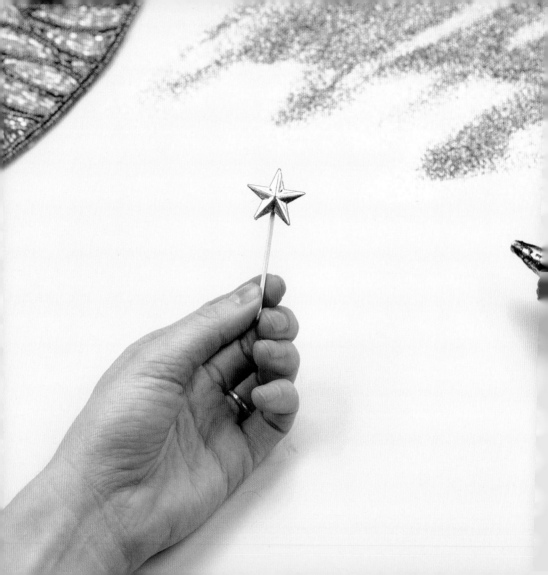

star pins

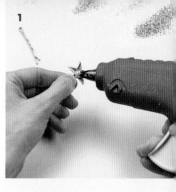

MATERIALS

hot glue gun • small star bead or stud •
conventional bobby pins to match your hair
color (or to match the color of the star)

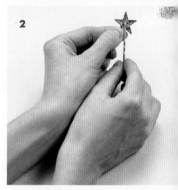

1. Apply a generous dot of hot glue to the back
of the star.

2. Press the flat side of the bobby pin loop into
the hot glue and allow to dry fully.

RESOURCES

Below are my favorite places to shop for all of my hair supplies. At these shops, you'll find everything you need to complete the styles in this book and to create your own pins. You may even be inspired to invent your own designs!

CRAFT SUPPLIES

ETSY.COM
An online resource for handmade crafts, clothes, art, beads, and much more. If you don't feel like making your own specialty pins, this is a great place to find lovely pins made by others.

MICHAELS CRAFT STORES
A great resource for any supplies you might need to make your own pins, such as glue, jewelry wire, and glitter, to name a few.

HAIR TOOLS AND PRODUCTS

SEPHORA
Traditionally a makeup store, you can also find a wide array of haircare products and tools here.

ULTA BEAUTY
A beauty superstore where you can purchase all haircare tools and products, as well as nail polish for painting your own pins.

ACKNOWLEDGMENTS

A very special thank-you to:

My agent, Adriann Ranta, for her endless guidance while this book came to fruition.

Chronicle Books, especially Laura Lee Mattingly, for giving me the opportunity to write my second book.

My friend and photographer, Justin Ouellette, for being easy and fun to work with and for taking the most beautiful photos.

Jen Dunlap, the best production designer, prop master, and artist in all the land—and my great friend.

Maryssa Stumpf, our amazing stylist.

Sarah Hall, for the beautiful makeup.

The models: Lizz Adams, Veronica Osario, Gabriela Lopez, Maryssa Stumpf, and Sarah Hall.

ModCloth for providing so many wardrobe pieces.

My family, for always believing in me.

Petunia, for sleeping under my desk and being my little companion while I wrote this book. You snore so loudly.

And last, but most, thank you to my husband, John. You are my best friend, my partner, my voice of reason, and my support. I cannot thank you enough for all your help during the making of this book, from keeping me company in my office while I wrote to holding reflectors during photo shoots. I'm so lucky, and I love every day with you.